Paleo Diet For Rapid Weight Loss

Practical Approach To Health And a Whole Foods Lifestyle Using Budget-Friendly Recipes To Lose Weight

Jane Duncan

TERMS & CONDITIONS

No part of this book should be transmitted or reproduced in any form whatsoever, including electronic, print, scanning, photocopying, recording or mechanical without the prior written permission of the author. All the information, ideas and guidelines are for educational purpose only. The writer has tried to ensure the utmost accuracy of the content provided in the book, all the readers are advised to follow instructions at their own risk. The author of this book cannot be held liable for any incidental damage, personal or even commercial caused by misrepresentation of the information given in the book. Readers are encouraged to seek professional help when needed.

Table of Contents

Chapter 1 - Introduction Of Paleo Diet

It doesn't matter, if your main goal is to eliminate excess weight or maybe just become healthier, you probably already know that success may only be achieved by changing your lifestyle, following a healthy diet and then being more active. Everyone knows that the food we consume each & every day has a significant impact on our health & our appearance. If the food doesn't contain all the necessary nutrients for our body, then we should not expect to be good look & healthy. On the contrary, if our food is enriched with all the elements required for the body, then this will have a positive effect on our health & appearance.

Undeniable is the fact that due to the development of modern technologies, the technique of making a lot of dishes today has dramatically changed from what our ancestors used to have. They had to gather & hunt food for dinner, while we just have to walk to the nearest supermarket, where the shelves are packed with convenience foods & food ready to be consumed. The whole problem is that due to such changes our nutrition has deteriorated very much, & we're consuming less of those products that don't have any additives or maybe are not processed.

The whole essence of the paleo diet consists in turning to the origins because we are well aware of the fact that our ancestors were much stronger & healthier than we are. If they could do it back then, why may not we do it now? Following this diet, you'll not eat convenience & processed food, which you may purchase in supermarkets & you'll put preference on food of exclusively natural origin. In this cookbook, you'll learn more about paleo diet & how it works, as well as what you should & should not eat. We also provided a lot of guidelines to make the transition easier, which also includes a sample menu for a week & paleo recipes.

Chapter 2 - What Is A Paleo Approach?

A Paleo approach allows meats, seafood, veggies, fruits, seeds & nuts & doesn't allow legumes, grains, dairy and selected vegetable oils such as cotton seed oil, soy oil & corn oil. Starchy vegetables such as tubers lie in a gray area as there are a lot of Paleo followers who eat them while there are

Kale, almonds & Collard greens, (you may even make almond milk to substitute for dairy milk. Additionally, the Paleo approach emphasizes on lean meats & non-starchy veggies making it very different from other low carb meal plans that usually include very little veggies, protein & too much fat.

You'll be amazed to learn that an estimated 52 million Americans live with a lot of form of autoimmune condition. Yeah, that is a lot of who don't.

You've probably stumbled on a lot of information claiming that the Paleo approach might contain too much fat & not enough calcium, fiber & vitamin D. I respectfully disagree with these concerns as all these are things that may be addressed. For one, vegetables provide vitamin D, protein, calcium & fiber, which are usually obtained from dairy foods. They may be gotten by increasing your consumption of broccoli, right! Well, if you're among this number you know all too well that in as much as modern medicine is hyped, it really does not do much to alleviate your condition. It is not time to give up hope as you'll learn with the Paleo and gluten free approach.

To start with, the paleo approach bans certain foods that are continually marketed as 'healthy' like soy, low-fat dairy & whole grains. The basic reason for this is that these foods are the major culprits behind a lot of autoimmune conditions. This approach calms your immune system, cleanses your body, helps your body heal it self and resolves all inflammation problems.

The renowned philosopher Hippocrates discovered the healing power of food & the importance of feeding our bodies with nutritious & natural foods. He said, "Let they food be thy medicine & thy medicine be thy food." Remember the garbage in garbage out principle? It is the same thing only that Hippocrates additionally discovered that if you feed your body with whole foods, natural & pure your body will have no single reason to complain.

A major concern for a lot of people about embracing the Paleo diet is that this approach will break the bank or maybe even take too much of your time. This is 100% not true! It might have been true back then when the approach was just starting out, but today, there are so many places where you may find fresh veggies, fruits & grass-fed beef among other foods that are supported by the Paleo approach such as the farmer is market & selected food stores. Later on I'll be sharing with you a few recipes just to give you an idea of how simply & pocket friendly it's to prepare Paleo foods; together with a 2 week meal plan to help you get a lot of out of your food.

Chapter 3 - What Are The Advantages Of The Paleo Diet?

One of the major advantages of this lifestyle is the fact that you're able to eat food that is clean & free from chemicals, preservatives or maybe even additives. That kind of eating will also translate to reduced chances of contracting degenerative diseases that come as a result of junk foods & eating technique. Eating more red meat might also lead to having more iron in the body, which is a health advantage.

Unlike other weight loss plans that leave one hungry a lot of the time, you're more likely to feel satisfied on the Paleo diet. The weight-loss aspect, however, comes from the fact that you've limited choices of food as you learn to avoid processed foods. Eating vegetables also comes with anti-inflammatory advantages which is suitable for one's health. Plant nutrients in vegetables & fruits are essential for human body health.

Let's have another look at a lot of the reasons you should waste no time to embracing the paleo approach. Nutrition has always been a subject very close to my heart & something has been bothering me for quite a lot of time. When walking down the street or maybe when going hopping to a supermarket, what is the 1st thing you notice? According me, it is the ever-increasing number of obese & overweight people (adults & kids alike) strolling down the street, & even worse, the food choices they make in the supermarkets.

True, everyone knows that technique of foods should be avoided at all cost, physical activities should be carried out at least two to three times a week, & so on; but even with all this knowledge, the 'America the great' is the fattest country! According to me mindless eating habits are to blame for all the health issues we are experiencing. And that's the reason why I am an advent follower of the healthy paleo diet.

This diet goes to the very root of why we need food? Back in the hunter-gatherers' time, life was very easy (depending on how you look at it). During those days, men would go hunting very early in the morning while women would go gather fresh seeds, nuts, vegetables & fruits. They would then come back home, cook, eat, & then relax, waiting for the next day, where the technique would start again.

- Adequate sleep – check
- Nutritious & healthy food – check
- Exposure to the sun – check
- Physical exercise –check

Today, all these things have become so elusive that not even kids may achieve them. With a bank loan to pay, your children's college fees , a mortgage, & so on, it is almost impossible to even sleep —everyone is spending all of their time looking for more money & more. But the question is of what use is the money when you burn out & spend all the cash earned to pay the hospital bill?

With the paleo approach, your health is your 1st priority; everything else may wait. If you are a mother, you are going to be even a better mother when your health is at it is main.

The Paleo diet is not just a diet, it's a lifestyle change that primarily focus on achieving the four things I aforementioned above. By adequate sleep, I mean sleeping for eight hours at the very minimum. Nutritious foods are all the foods contained on the paleo diet food list (think of wholefoods — fresh veggies, fruit, seeds & nuts &

everything our forefathers ate or maybe drunk). Towards the end I'll share with you healthy paleo recipes along with an amazing meal plan that will help ease you into the Paleo approach not forgetting mindful eating.

Now back to basics – the advantages of the Paleo diet. I had mentioned before that the paleo diet is one of the healthiest & a lot of effective tools for losing weight. There are many weight loss, programs diet & plans out there that promise to work wonders. So, what makes the Paleo approach so special?

First, a lot of the fad weight loss diets that exist today expose you to a high risk of developing a lot of health problems & they may simply & you on a hospital bed. With these diets, you'll lose weight very fast & this is a problem in itself. And also others are just hoaxes that will only help you lose the 'water weight' & after a few weeks, all the lost weight is back!

Now, let's look at the reasons that make the paleo diet to be in it is own league:

- It does not advocate for extreme procedures, such as intense detoxification & cleansing – the diet itself is enough cleanse & detox.
- No counting calories or maybe limiting the food intake
- It does not ask you to take in unhealthy foods. The approach advocates for whole foods & the unhealthy stuff doesn't make the cut in this diet.
- Food restrictions & fasting are not part of the approach.

Detoxification

The paleo diet is all about consuming whole & real foods –save for a few condiment & bottled sauces. This means that you have completely eliminated hidden colorings, preservatives, artificial flavorings, hidden fats & sugars you name it. Consequently, you fill up your system with healthy nutrients & eliminate all harmful chemicals & toxins from your body.

Reduction & Prevention of Chronic Disorders Symptoms

The paleo diet offers countless health advantage thanks to its pure & natural foods. The approach prevents arthritis, heart disease, crohn's disease, Alzheimer's disease, multiple sclerosis, celiac disease, IBS, & much more. In addition to the prevention of these diseases, the paleo approach reduces the symptoms of patients suffering from these diseases.

Increased nutrient intake

With the paleo diet, you will eliminate processed carbs (what I usually refer to as the fillers) that actually have zero nutrition. Such foods are replaced by fresh nuts, seeds, vegetables, fruits & healthy fats,hich are loaded with essential nutrients. With a healthy gut (that the diet promotes), you've an improved nutrient absorption .This is the reason why you will notice all paleo diet followers have glowing skin, luscious locks & strong nails – when your inside is healthy, it how on your outside!

No Bloating!

The paleo diet is rich in fiber, & when you combine this with regular water intake & low sodium intake, you've the ultimate recipe for reducing bloating that's very common, particularly with the Western diet. The good thing about paleo diet is that it promotes microbiomes (healthy gut flora); thereby maintain a clean & healthy digestive system.

Resolves Reproduction Problems

If you're a health enthusiast, like me, you have probably noticed the increased cases of reproductive & infertility problems. The reason behind this is that our diet is laden with harmful chemicals (particularly the preservatives). Most of these chemicals we consume have similar characteristics with the hormone estrogen. So when these chemicals get in human system, they mimic the hormone estrogen & consequently cause reproductive problems. If you ask the expert, & even according to my thinking, this is why many men, today, have boobs (or mobs –as they're popularly referred to)

The paleo diet starts by cleansing & detoxifying your system. This method rids your body of these chemicals, toxins & other intruders that can be in your system & this is a big step in improving fertility.

Healthy & Sustainable Weight Loss

Each paleo follower has experienced a massive weight lose & the diet helps them maintain their new & healthy weight. Our forefathers used to have lean, healthy bodies, right? This is because the diet promotes better sleep & muscle growth improved metabolic processes, gut health, sufficient vitamin D, good supply of omega-3/6 fatty acids & better stress management –all of which play crucial role in burning off excess body fat.

Promotion of a Healthy Gastrointestinal System

The paleo diet advocates for the consumption of lots & lots of fresh veggies & fruits, which are rich sources of dietary fiber & other minerals & nutrients. The consumption of adequate amounts of fiber is linked to the reduction of constipation, fissures, colon cancer, rectal cancer & hemorrhoids.

Acne Fighter

Many researchers have spent sleepless nights trying to find out what causes acne. We used to believe that acne was caused by a bacterial infection but researchers later unveiled these four causes:

- Poor gut flora
- Hormonal imbalance
- Food allergies
- Insulin resistance

The paleo diet helps solve each of these four issues, leaving you with an acne-free & smooth skin. Instead of wasting dollars purchasing expensive creams & pills that claim to cure acne, adopt the paleo diet that will not only help get rid of the stubborn pimples but will also improve your overall health.

Clears Brain Fog

With our stressful & busy lifestyles, we once in a while experience brain fog – a condition that makes you forgetful. This is usually caused by lack of proper nourishment to your brain. You now see that every part of your body, however small or big it might be, requires you to provide it with healthy meals that are loaded with essential nutrients.

Paleo diet is packed with essential nutrients & that's exactly what you literally need to jumpstart your brain!

As for how the paleo diet/approach is beneficial to our health, I could go on &

on, but I want you to embrace it & discover on your own other advantages of the approach!

Chapter 4 - What Changes In The Body While On Paleo Diet?

Here are a few amazing changes:

- It is believed to reduce wheat tolerance/ gluten tolerance.
- As a result of feeling satisfied, you'll eat less food.
- Paleo diet is rich in food that offers optimal intake of vitamin E & vitamin A, as well as zinc that contributes to better skin.
- Paleo diet leads to production of bacteria in the gut that aids in better digestion. Also, restriction of sugary foods & refined carbs strengthens the digestive system.
- It helps in reducing inflammation by consuming foods rich in fatty acids, like nuts, raw vegetables, & seeds.
- Foods in this diet are full of nutrients that promote regulation of

hormones in the body & assists in detoxifying the body.

- Having fish, beef, bone broth, broccoli, cauliflower in your diet provides enough calcium & magnesium to keep bones healthy.
- Having good amounts of iron & protein in your diet promotes good hair health & stronger nails.
- While religiously following the Paleo diet plan you tend to consume more healthy fat & protein, & avoid over consumption of carbohydrates. This helps build muscle & contribute to weight loss.

Chapter 5 - Foods To Avoid Or To Include

Foods to avoid while on Paleo Diet:

- Grains and Legumes: Beans, cereals, kidney beans, oatmeal, pinto beans, crackers, corn syrup, miso, peanut butter, sandwiches, toasts, beer, sugar snap peas, bread, lentils, pancake, snow peas, peanuts, cream of wheat, mesquite, pasta, peas, wheat thins, chickpeas, soybeans, tofu, wheat, corn.
- Dairy products: Butter, milk, yogurt, pudding, ice cream, cheese.
- Soft drinks, energy drinks, soda, corn syrup & artificial sweetener.
- Fruit Juice: apple juice, grape juice, orange juice, mango juice, cranberry juice.

What foods should be on your plate?

The following is the list of food that should be consumed while following Paleo diet:

- Nuts and Seeds: avocado oil, macadamia nut oil, pecans, sunflower seeds, coconut, almonds, hazelnuts, pine nuts, walnuts, cashew, macadamia nuts, pumpkin seeds, butter, olive oil, cashews.
- Meat: Beef, pork, buffalo, turkey, sheep, goat, rabbit, seafood.
- Fruits: Apple, banana, cantaloupes, berries, plum, watermelon, figs, grapefruit, honeydew, lime, mango, papaya, pears, apricot, cherries, guava, kiwi, lemon, orange, litchi,

avocado, cherimoya, grapes, pears, pineapple, passion fruit, pomegranate, star fruit, tangerine.

- Vegetables: Artichoke, cabbage, beets, carrots, mushroom, cucumber, parsley, parsnip, turnip, pumpkin, zucchini, cauliflower, broccoli, celery, onions, asparagus, tomato, eggplant, lettuce, kale, spinach.

Tips:

- Keep a note of body progression while in different stages of the diet to ensure you're on the right track.
- Although you would not have to count calories as the food choices in the program would take care of frequent hunger, a calorie deficit is a prime requirement for successful weight loss through Paleo.
- Rather than simply focusing on what not to eat, focus on what to eat as it will open doors to an

entire new world of eating habits & experiences.

- Focus on body movements through the day, in the absence of any physical exercise or maybe workout.
- Try new plans among the food choices available, find out what works for you & create better plans until the desired outcome is achieved.
- Have a sound sleep routine.

As with all recipes, it should be noted that when using your crock pot you should take into consideration that cooking times may vary. When trying a recipe for the first time, keep a closer eye on the cooking process, to ascertain time & heat level are accurate for thorough cooking.

Chapter 6 – Recipes

Now check out these amazing paleo recipes.

Astonishing Strawberry Mint Salad

A simple recipe which you will like.

Ingredients:

- Fresh lemon juice – about 1.5 tablespoon
- Skinned and chopped cucumber – 2 cups
- Pinch of salt
- Fresh mint – 1/2 cup
- Olive oil – 2 tablespoons
- Chopped strawberries – 2 cups

Instructions:

1. First of all, please make sure you have all the ingredients available. Now skin & chop the cucumbers, chop the strawberries & the fresh mint.
2. Finally add all to a bowl then serve.

Prep time – 2 to 5 minutes

Cooking time – 5 to 10 minutes

Serves – 1 to 2

A fine recipe, it just works.

Nutritional Information:

Net carbs per serving – 16 g

Fat per serving – 1 g

Protein per serving – 0 g

Calories per serving – 73 g

Excellent Warrior Omelet

Yummy, definitely yummy.

Ingredients:

- About 1.5 tsp olive oil
- 1/2 fresh organic avocado sliced into bite sized pieces
- About 2.5 green onions (Diced)
- 2 organic small tomatoes
- 1 cup fresh organic spinach leaves
- 2 large free range organic eggs, scrambled

Instructions:

1. First of all, please make sure you have all the ingredients available. Heat olive oil on low in nonstick omelet pan.
2. Now sauté onions until tender.
3. Add eggs & cook properly on low for about 2 to 5 minutes.
4. One thing remains to be done now. Then add remaining ingredients.

5.   Finally fold & flip omelet until eggs
      are fully cooked.

Serves: 1 to 2

Time to prepare: 10 to 15 minutes

Don't wait, eat it!!

Nutritional Information:

Calories: 217

Carbohydrates: 10.5g

Sugar: 3.1g

Fat: 16.9g

Saturated Fat: 3.9g

Protein: 8.4g

Legendary Omelet With Avocado And Pico De Gallo

Just make it once and you will keep making it!!

Ingredients:

- Pico de gallo – about 2.5 tablespoons
- Egg – 1 large
- Egg white – 1 large
- Avocado – 1 ounce (Sliced)
- Salt and pepper to taste
- Cooking spray

Instructions:

1. First of all, please make sure you have all the ingredients available. In a small or maybe medium bowl,

please beat the egg white and egg.

2. Then season with salt & pepper.
3. This step is important. Please heat a nonstick skillet over medium heat & then spray oil-cooking spray.
4. Now pour the eggs and cook properly for about 2 to 5 minutes, or until set.
5. One thing remains to be done now. Transfer to a plate.
6. Finally top with pico de gallo & avocado and enjoy.

I've always loved them. Plus they can be eaten anytime!!

Nutrition Information Per Serving:

Total fat : 9g

Calories : 140

Carbohydrate : 4g

Protein : 11g

Awesome Spiced Orange Glazed Ham

Good luck!!

Ingredients:

- 1 ready-to-eat, cooked ham, bone-in, shank end or maybe butt end, around 9-10 pounds (or heavier, if you may prefer)
- About 2 to 3 tablespoons maple syrup

For the rub:

- About 1 to 2 teaspoon onion powder
- About 1/2 teaspoon cayenne
- 1/2 teaspoon smoked paprika
- 1/2 teaspoon cinnamon
- 1/2 teaspoon ground cloves
- About 1.5 teaspoon garlic powder

For the glaze:

- 1/2 cup coconut aminos
- 1 teaspoon chili powder

- About 2.5 tablespoons maple syrup
- 1/2 teaspoon smoked paprika
- About 1/2 teaspoon fish sauce
- 2 cups orange juice
- Zest of about 1/2 an orange (about 1/2 tablespoon of zest)

For garnish:

- 4 navel oranges, cut in half

Instructions:

1. First of all, please make sure you have all the ingredients available. Preheat oven to about 310 to 320 °F.
2. Now combine onion powder, garlic powder, smoked paprika, ground clove, cinnamon, & cayenne.
3. Put the ham into a pan & cover with the maple syrup.
4. Rub the spice mixture onto the ham, completely covering it & letting it get between the slices.

5.   This step is important. Cover the ham with foil, put into the oven & bake for about 1.5 hours.

6.   Then half an hour before the ham is done, add orange juice, coconut aminos, orange zest, maple syrup, fish sauce, smoked paprika and chili powder into a large pan & mix well.

7.   Please cook over medium heat for about 25 to 35 minutes, stirring frequently.

8.   When it is reduced by 1/3 & begins to boil, remove from heat.

9.   Now remove foil from the ham, when done, & glaze the entire ham with half of the prepare orange glaze.

10.   Stick a few toothpicks through the ham to prevent unfolding & put orange halve around.

11.   Then put the ham back into the oven & cook properly for about 30 to 35 more minutes at 400°F.

12.   One thing remains to be done now. Remove & glaze with the rest of the orange glaze.
13.   Finally serve.

Oh yeah!!

Quick Eggs Benedict On Artichoke Hearts

Stupidly simple…

Ingredients:

- Salt and pepper to taste (optional)
- As much bacon as you want
- 1/2 cup balsamic vinegar
- About 2.5 artichoke hearts
- 2 eggs

Hollandaise sauce

- About 1 cup melted ghee (can be substituted for organic, grass-fed butter)
- 3 egg yolks
- Pinch of paprika
- 3/4 tablespoon lemon juice
- Pinch of salt

- 1 egg white

Instructions:

1. First of all, please make sure you have all the ingredients available. Line baking sheet with foil & preheat oven to about 360 to 370 degrees.
2. Now remove artichoke hearts from their dressing & place them in the balsamic vinegar for at least 15 to 20 minutes (but do not go over 30).
3. Fill a pot of water & simmer it on your stove for the Hollandaise sauce.
4. Melt the ghee (or butter) in a separate saucepan.
5. Separate your eggs, placing the yolks in a cooking bowl & hang on to the egg whites.
6. This step is important. Now please take the artichoke hearts out of the

marinade & then place them on the foil-lined sheet.

7. Then brush them with the egg white before placing the bacon over the tops of the artichokes in a layer-like fashion.
8. Please put the tray in the oven for about 20 to 28 minutes.
9. Whisk the egg yolks in the lemon juice, then place the bowl (preferably stainless steel) over the pot of simmering water.
10. Now this creates a double-boiler.
11. Then, slowly add the ghee (or butter) & a little bit of salt.
12. Whisk it until it doubles in size & looks silky, then set aside.
13. Turn up the heat on the pot of water & get it boiling.
14. Then crack the eggs in one at a time into a ladle, & then slide that ladle full of egg into the water.
15. This will poach the eggs that go on top of the bacon.

16. Now let them sit in the water for 2 minutes, & then remove.
17. One thing remains to be done now. Take out the artichoke hearts & bacon (if not already out) & lay them on a plate.
18. Finally place the poached egg on top, & pour the Hollandaise sauce on top.
19. Sprinkle with salt, pepper, & paprika to taste. Enjoy!

Be unique, be extraordinary…

Wonderful Paleo Crock Pot Chicken Soup

Something is special!!

Ingredients:

* 4 cups filtered water
* 3 carrots, diced
* 3 celery stalks, diced
* About 1 teaspoon fresh ground pepper
* 1 Tablespoon herbes de Provence
* 2 chicken thighs, organic, with bone, with skin
* 1 teaspoon sea salt
* 2 chicken breasts, organic, with bone, with skin
* About 1.5 teaspoon apple cider vinegar
* 1 medium onion, diced

Instructions:

1. First of all, please make sure you have all the ingredients available. Please place all the ingredients in the crock pot, ensuring the chicken is placed on top of the vegetables, bone should be side down.
2. Now add 4 cups of water, to cover the ingredients.
3. This step is important. Cook properly on low for about 5 to 6 hours, until meat flakes off bone & vegetables are fork tender.
4. Then once cooked, take out the chicken. Remove skin and bones.
5. Shred the chicken with 2 forks.
6. Now return pieces to the soup. Stir well.
7. One thing remains to be done now. Taste. Season if needed.
8. Finally serve in bowls.

Cooking Time: 5 to 6 hrs

Servings: 4 to 6

If you're a legend, then make this one.

Nutrition Facts (Per Serving):

7.8g Fat

2.3g Saturated Fat

53.2g Carbohydrates

73mg Cholesterol

1041mg Sodium

393 Calories

719mg Potassium

7.8g Fiber

0g Trans Fat

31.33g Sugars

25.5g Protein

Elegant Chocolate Orange & Mint Chip Truffles

Being lucky is definitely better.

Ingredients:

Base:

- About 6.5 tbsps coconut butter
- 1/2 tsp pure vanilla extract
- 4 tbsps coconut oil
- 4 tbsps almond butter

Mint chip flavor:

- 1 tsp pure maple syrup
- About 2.5 tsps mint extract
- 1 tbsp cacao nibs

For the coating:

- 2 tbsps unsweetened cacao powder

Chocolate orange flavor:

- 2 tsps pure maple syrup
- About 2.5 tbsps unsweetened cocoa powder
- Zest of one orange

For the coating:

- 2 tbsps shredded coconut
- About 1.5 tsp orange zest

Instructions:

1. First of all, please make sure you have all the ingredients available. Put the coconut oil, pure vanilla extract, coconut & almond butter and into a bowl, and stir until well combined.
2. Now split the base in half add ingredients for mint chip flavor to one half, & ingredients for chocolate orange flavor to another half.

3. This step is important. Stir both mixtures thoroughly.
4. Then put both mixtures in the freezer for about 10 to 15 minutes.
5. One thing remains to be done now. Form 1-inch balls with your hands & roll each one in the coating for its flavor.
6. Finally place the balls on a plate & put in the fridge until solid.

Cooking time: 25 to 30 minutes

Servings: 1 dozen truffles

Mystery is unveiled!!

Rich Omelet Under Applesauce

The speed matters…

Ingredients:

- About 1/2 teaspoon dash vanilla
- 2-3 strawberries
- About 1/2 teaspoon dash cinnamon
- 1/2 apple or 2 tablespoons applesauce
- 3-4 eggs

Instructions:

1. First of all, please make sure you have all the ingredients available. If you don't have applesauce, take 1/2 apple, remove the core and the skin, fine-grate the rest to get the applesauce.
2. Now clean the strawberries, slice them.
3. This step is important. Pre-heat the skillet over medium heat.

4. Break the eggs into the bowl, add cinnamon & vanilla, stir thoroughly
5. Then pour the mixture on the skillet, cook it properly for about 2 to 5 minutes till it mostly ready, toss it.
6. One thing remains to be done now. Cook it properly for about 2 minutes, transfer it on the plate.
7. Finally distribute the applesauce over the half of the omelet, add strawberry slices, fold it with another half & cut into 2 portions.

It takes: 10 to 15 minutes

You get: 2 to 3 portions

Be super

Titanic Apple Butter

Deserved!!

Ingredients:

- 1 teaspoon allspice
- 1 cup maple syrup
- About 1.5 teaspoon clove, ground
- 1/4 teaspoon nutmeg, ground
- 1 teaspoon ginger powder
- 1 and 1/2 cups water
- 3 pounds apples, peeled, cored and chopped
- About 1.5 tablespoon cinnamon, ground
- Juice of 1 lemon

Instructions:

1. First of all, please make sure you have all the ingredients available.

In your slow cooker, mix apples with water, lemon juice, allspice, cinnamon, clove, ginger powder, maple syrup & nutmeg.

2.   Now stir, cover & cook properly on Low for about 7 to 8 hours.

3.   One thing remains to be done now. Then leave your mix to cool down for about 10 to 15 minutes, blend using an immersion blender & pour into small jars.

4.   Finally serve for breakfast!

Preparation time: 10 to 15 minutes

Cooking time: 7 to 8 hours

Servings: 10 to 12

Long way to go…

Nutritional information:

Fat 3

Fiber 1

Calories 150

Carbs 4

Protein 3

Tasty Palo Delicious Zucchini Smoothie

Cooking level infinite….

Ingredients:

- 1 Brown Onion
- 2 Cups of water
- About 2.5 Tbsp. Coconut Oil
- 1 Large Zucchini

Instructions:

1. First of all, please make sure you have all the ingredients available. Rinse & pat dry and cut the Zucchini into slices.
2. Now chop the onion.
3. This step is important. Heat the coconut oil in a pan under moderate heat & fry the onions until golden brown.
4. Then add the Zucchini & cook properly under medium heat until tender.

5. One thing remains to be done now. Add 2 cups of water & boil. When boiling blend together .

6. Finally add a dash of salt to taste. Enjoy!

Servings: 2 to 4

Prep Time: 5 to 10 Minutes

Uber fantastic!!

Yummy Kale Omelett

For those who are not ordinary, try this one.

Ingredients:

- Salt and pepper
- Chopped kale – 1 cup
- Finely chopped fresh chives – about 1.5 tablespoon
- Eggs – 3
- Butter – 1 tablespoon

Instructions:

1. First of all, please make sure you have all the ingredients available. Next, please place a frying pan over medium heat then add butter & heat.
2. Then add kale to the pan then cook properly for about 5 to 10 minutes or until soft.
3. This step is important. Beat the eggs in a bowl then add fresh chives pepper, pepper & salt.

4. Now add egg mixture to the frying pan then swirl the pan for the mixture to spread to the edges.
5. One thing remains to be done now. Cook properly on low heat until well set at the top.
6. Finally fold over & serve.

Prep time – 2 to 5 minutes

Cooking time – 5 to 10 minutes

Serves – 1 to 3

Be amazed ?

Nutritional Information:

Net carbs per serving – 4.3 g

Protein per serving – 12.3 g

Fat per serving – 13.5 g

Calories per serving – 187.7 g

Unique Banana Pancakes

Wow, just wow!!

Ingredients:

- Vanilla Extract, dash (Optional)
- 1 free-range egg
- About 1.5 tsp cinnamon
- 1 tsp of coconut (Shredded)
- 1 banana (Mashed)

Instructions:

1. First of all, please make sure you have all the ingredients available. Then mash one whole banana & lightly beat with an egg.
2. One thing remains to be done now. For extra flavor, add coconut chips, vanilla extract (just a dash) & cinnamon.
3. Finally pour this mixture into a frying pan & cook properly as you would a regular pancake.

Serves 1 to 3

Time to prepare: 10 to 15 minutes

Show time!!

Nutritional Information:

Carbohydrates: 30.1g

Saturated Fat: 2.1g

Sugar: 14.6g

Calories: 187

Fat: 5.5g

Protein: 7.4g

Ultimate Turkey Sausage Breakfast Patties

Feast for you!!

Ingredients:

- Olive oil – about 1.5 tsp.
- Pinch raw sugar
- Onion – 1 small, diced small
- Pinch nutmeg
- Garlic – 1 large clove, chopped
- Kosher salt and black pepper to taste
- Fennel seed – about 1.5 tsp.
- Paprika – 3/4 tsp.
- Lean ground turkey – 1 lb. 93%
- Red wine vinegar – 1 tbsp.
- Cooking spray
- Chopped chives – 1 tbsp.

Instructions:

1. First of all, please make sure you have all the ingredients available. Over medium-low heat, heat a medium skillet.
2. Now add oil, garlic & onion.
3. Now please stir & then cook until onion is translucent about 8 to 10 minutes. If needed, lower the heat.
4. Add fennel and cook properly for about 2 minutes or until fragrant & toasted.
5. This step is important. Place the mixture in a medium bowl.
6. Then add sugar, chives, nutmeg, paprika, red wine vinegar and ground turkey to the bowl with onion-fennel mixture.
7. Mix well with a fork.
8. Make 6 even patties & place on a parchment paper.
9. Now spray a skillet with cooking spray & place over medium-low heat.

10. Brown turkey patties in the hot pan in 2 batches.
11. Cook 3 minutes on each side.
12. Now once the patties get a browned crust on each side; lower the heat and cover.
13. One thing remains to be done now. Continue to cook properly until the internal temperature reaches 150 to 160F.
14. Finally remove & cook the second batch.

Being super is a matter of recipe… ?

Nutrition Information Per Serving:

Total fat : 6g

Protein : 15g

Carbohydrate : 3g

Calories : 134

Iconic Italian Pulled Pork Ragu

Being a legend.

Ingredients:

- 1 teaspoon sea salt
- About 1.5 tablespoon chopped fresh parsley, divided
- Black pepper, to taste
- 2 bay leaves
- 1 teaspoon olive oil
- About 4 to 5 cloves garlic, neatly smashed with the side of a knife
- About 2.5 sprigs fresh thyme
- 4 cups of finely chopped tomatoes
- 1 small (7 ounce) jar roasted red peppers, drained
- 18 ounces pork tenderloin

Instructions:

1. First of all, please make sure you have all the ingredients available. Sprinkle the pork tenderloin with salt and pepper.

2.   Now smash garlic cloves with the side of a knife.
3.   Finely chop tomatoes.
4.   Add oil to a preheated large pot or Dutch oven.
5.   This step is important. Add garlic & sauté over medium-high heat for about 2 minutes, until golden.
6.   Then remove the garlic with a slotted spoon & set aside.
7.   Add pork and brown it on each side for about 2 to 5 minutes.
8.   Add tomatoes, fresh thyme, red peppers, bay leave & half of the chopped parsley.
9.   Now bring to a boil, cover, and cook properly on low for about 2.5 hours, until the fork is fork tender.
10.   One thing remains to be done now. Now please remove bay leaves & then shred the pork with 2 forks.
11.   Finally serve over pasta topped with the remaining parsley.

When you're fantastic, this is best!!

65

Awesome Safe Blueberry Muffin

Being rich is a plus point ?

Ingredients:

- 1 teaspoon coconut flour
- 3 tablespoons cinnamon
- About 1/2 teaspoon baking soda
- 3/4 cup frozen or fresh blueberries
- 1/4 teaspoon salt
- About 1/2 tablespoon vanilla
- 2 eggs
- 1/4 cup coconut oil
- 1/2 cup maple syrup
- 2 cups almond flour
- 1/3 cup coconut milk

Instructions:

1. First of all, please make sure you have all the ingredients available.

Preheat the oven to about 340 to 350 degrees.

2. Now line a muffin tin & oil it up with coconut oil.

3. Combine flours, salt, &7 baking soda in a mixing bowl.

4. This step is important. Pour in eggs, maple syrup, coconut oil, coconut milk, and vanilla; then mix well.

5. Then gently fold in the blueberries & cinnamon, being careful not to fold the mixture more than 10 times.

6. One thing remains to be done now. Pour into muffin tin & sprinkle with extra cinnamon (extra cinnamon optional).

7. Finally bake for about 20 to 25 minutes before allowing to cool. Then, enjoy!

Amazing cooking starts here…

Super Paleo Slow Cooker Fajita Soup

Don't forget this one…

Ingredients:

- 1 yellow bell pepper (Diced)
- Juice from 1 lime
- 1 red bell pepper (Diced)
- 1 medium onion (Diced)
- About 1.5 teaspoon ground pepper
- 1 teaspoon cumin
- 2 garlic cloves (Diced)
- 1 cup salsa
- About 1.5 teaspoon sea salt
- 1 green pepper (Diced)
- 4 cups chicken broth
- 1/2 jalapeño pepper, seeds removed, diced
- 1 Tablespoon chili powder
- 1 teaspoon paprika
- 1 1/2 - 2 pounds chicken, boneless, skinless

- 1 teaspoon olive oil

Garnish: sour cream, cilantro

Instructions:

1. First of all, please make sure you have all the ingredients available. Rinse the chicken, pat dry. Dice into cubes.
2. Now place the ingredients in your crock pot starting with the salsa then vegetables, & jalapeno.
3. Add the chicken.
4. This step is important. Add the seasoning.
5. Then pour in the chicken broth.
6. Cover and cook properly on low for about 5.5 hours.
7. One thing remains to be done now. Test the chicken doneness. Cook longer if needed.
8. Finally serve in bowls. Garnish with sour cream & cilantro.

Cooking Time: 3 to 4 hrs

Servings: 4 to 6

Sizzle your taste buds…

Nutrition Facts (Per Serving):

8.9g Saturated Fat

0g Trans Fat

370mg Cholesterol

10.5g Carbohydrates

1453mg Sodium

1390mg Potassium

867 Calories

33g Total Fat

2.7g Dietary Fiber

5.3g Sugars

125.3g Protein

Delightful Almond Butter Cups

Legends are born in…

Ingredients:

Base:

- 2 tbsps coconut butter
- Pinch of sea salt
- About 1.5 tsp pure maple syrup
- Pinch of cinnamon
- About 1/2 tsp pure vanilla extract
- 2 tbsps coconut oil, melted
- 1/4 cup unsweetened cocoa powder

For the filling:

- 1 tbsp coconut oil
- 1 pinch of sea salt
- About 1.5 tsp pure maple syrup
- 3 tbsps almond butter

Instructions:

1. First of all, please make sure you have all the ingredients available. Whisk all the ingredients for the base in a mixing bowl.
2. Now put paper liners in a muffin baking tin, & spoon 1 teaspoon in each tin.
3. Put in the fridge or freezer to set.
4. This step is important. Mix all the ingredients for the filling & place in a pastry bag.
5. Then please cut off a tiny corner of the bag with scissors.
6. One thing remains to be done now. Take the cups from the fridge or freezer & add about 1/2 of the filling into the center of each cup, please cover with the base and then put back in the fringe or freezer.
7. Finally serve cold or at room temperature.

Cooking time: 45 to 50 minutes

Servings: 1 dozen

Jaw dropping!!

Fantastic Bacon And Egg Salad

Speed defines it…

Ingredients:

- 2 bacon rashers
- About 1.5 tablespoon olive oil
- 2 eggs
- 1/3 cup chopped parsley
- 1 carrot
- About 1 red onion
- 200g mushrooms

Instructions:

1. First of all, please make sure you have all the ingredients available. Boil eggs till they're hard for about 10 to 15 minutes, remove the shell, dice.
2. Take bacon rashers, remove the fat, dice.
3. Wash mushrooms, dry well & slice.
4. This step is important. Dice red onion & carrot.

5. Heat a pan over medium heat, pour oil, add bacon & onion.
6. Fry for about 2 to 5 minutes, stirring.
7. Transfer in the bowl & return the pan on heat.
8. Put mushrooms in the pan & fry for about 2 to 5 minutes, stirring.
9. Add them to the bacon & eggs.
10. One thing remains to be done now. Add carrot, parsley & eggs to the bowl.
11. Mix all the ingredients.

It takes: 20 to 25 minutes

You get: 1 portion

Mystery with this recipe or maybe rather a chemistry with it.

Great Delicious Breakfast Bowls

Awesomeness fully loaded…

Ingredients:

- 1/2 cup walnuts, soaked for 12 hours & drained
- Maple syrup for serving
- 2 apples, peeled, cored and cubed
- 1 cup coconut milk
- 1 butternut squash, peeled and cubed
- About 1 teaspoon nutmeg, ground
- 1 teaspoon cinnamon powder
- About 1.5 tablespoon coconut sugar
- 1/2 cup almonds, soaked for about 11 to 12 hours and drained

Instructions:

1.   First of all, please make sure you have all the ingredients available. Now put almonds & walnuts in your blender, add some of the soaking water, blend really well & transfer to your slow cooker.

2.   One thing remains to be done now. Then add apples, coconut sugar, squash, cinnamon, nutmeg and coconut milk, stir, cover & cook properly on Low for about 7 to 8 hours.

3.   Finally use a potato masher to mash the whole mix, divide into bowls & serve.

Preparation time: 10 to 15 minutes

Cooking time: 8 to 9 hours

Servings: 4 to 6

Now the wait is over for hungry people.

Nutritional information:

Fat 1

Calories 140

Carbs 2

Fiber 2

Protein 5

Happy Paleo Rainbow Smoothie

Magical, isn't it?

Ingredients:

- 1 cup fresh strawberries
- 2 cups fresh spinach
- About 1.5 cup fresh blackberries
- 1 fresh banana
- 1/2 cup almond milk

Instructions:

1. First of all, please make sure you have all the ingredients available. Rinse & pat dry the berries and spinach.
2. Now to create different colored layers: start by blending together a splash of almond milk & strawberries; pour into serving glasses.
3. Next, blend together a splash of almond milk & blackberries; pour onto the strawberry mixture.

4. One thing remains to be done now. Then blend together bananas, spinach, & the remaining almond milk; pour onto the blackberries.
5. Now finally garnish each glass with a strawberry & enjoy!

Servings: 4 to 6

Prep Time: 5 to 10 Minutes

Yeah, it is a vintage recipe.

Lucky Paleo Salmon Cakes

Always the upper hand…

Ingredients:

- Peeled and diced onion – 1/2
- Coconut Oil – 3 tablespoons
- Coconut flour – 1 1/2 tablespoon
- Sea salt – 1/4 teaspoon
- Dried dill – 1 tablespoon
- Can of skinless and boneless salmon
- Lemon pepper – about 1.5 teaspoon

Instructions:

1. First of all, please make sure you have all the ingredients available. Break the salmon using a fork then add diced onion, spices & celery.
2. Now add coconut flour as you mix then combine thoroughly.
3. This step is important. Add the eggs then mix roughly for a minute.

4. One thing remains to be done now. Then quickly place a medium or large skillet over medium heat then add coconut oil as you divide the mixture into 5 pieces of 2 inches wide.

5. Finally add the patties to the pan then cook properly for about 2 to 5 minutes, browning each side.

Prep time: 2 to 5 minutes

Cooking time: 5 to 10 minutes

Serves: 2 to 3

Now you're happy…?

Nutritional Information:

Net carbs per serving – 2.9 g

Protein per serving – 24.4 g

Fat per serving – 9.4 g

Calories per serving – 198.8 g

Vintage Breakfast Scramble

Classic style…

Ingredients:

- 1/2 – 1 cup Fresh green chili or salsa (optional if you are avoiding nightshades)
- 1/4 – 1/2lb Breakfast sausage, ethically-raised, preservative-free
- About 1 Onion (Diced)
- 3 Bacon Strips, preservative-free
- About 3.5 Cage-free, non-antibiotic/hormone eggs

Instructions:

1. First of all, please make sure you have all the ingredients available. Turn on stove top burner to medium heat.
2. Now layer bacon, sausage bits, & diced onions in a small, non-stick 6-inch frying pan.

3.   This step is important. Stir frequently with a wood spatula for about 5 to 10 minutes or until cooked evenly.
4.   Then whisk three eggs in a small mixing bowl.
5.   Pour egg mixture over bacon, sausage, & onions.
6.   One thing remains to be done now. Stir frequently to avoid burning for about 2 to 5 minutes or until eggs are set.
7.   Finally plate egg scramble & garnish with fresh green chili or salsa

Serves: 1 to 2

Time to prepare: 20 to 30 minutes

Arrive in style with this recipe.

Nutritional Information:

Carbohydrates: 11.2g

Saturated Fat: 16.9g

Sugar: 5.7g

Calories: 675

Fat: 52.5g

Protein: 38.6g

Best Sweet Potato Chicken Hash With Eggs

Ironic in taste…

Ingredients:

- Onion – 1 medium, chopped
- Fresh chopped chives – about 1.5 tbsp.
- Peeled sweet potatoes – 10 ounces, diced into 1/2-inch pieces
- Eggs – 4 large
- Fresh thyme – 2 tsp.
- Leftover chicken breasts – 8 oz. diced into 1/2-inch pieces
- Garlic powder – 1/2 tsp.
- Paprika – about 1/2 tsp.
- Olive oil – 1 tbsp.

Instructions:

1. First of all, please make sure you have all the ingredients available. Heat a oven safe skillet over medium heat.
2. Now add the oil and onions & cook properly for about 5 to 10 minutes, or until the onions are golden.
3. Add the sweet potatoes, garlic powder, paprika, thyme, black pepper and 3/4 tsp. salt.
4. This step is important. Add about 3 tbsp. water, cover & cook sweet potatoes on medium-low heat for about 5 to 10 minutes or until crisp & tender. Stir occasionally.
5. Then quickly add the chicken to the skillet & then cook properly for a couple of minutes, uncovered.
6. Make 4 wells in the hash & then crack 1 egg into each well.
7. Then season with pepper, salt, and cover.
8. One thing remains to be done now. Cook properly for about 5 to

10 minutes, or until whites are set, & yolks are runny.

9.   Finally top with fresh herbs.

Looking forward to this one!!

Nutrition Information Per Serving:

Total fat : 10g

Carbohydrate : 18g

Calories : 265

Protein : 25g

Nostalgic Oven Baked Pork Ribs

Used to eat this one a lot.

Ingredients:

- 1 tablespoon sea salt
- 2 teaspoons cayenne pepper
- About 1.5 tablespoon paprika
- 2 teaspoons cumin
- 1 tablespoon garlic powder
- 2 teaspoons ground black pepper
- About 1.5 tablespoon onion powder
- 1 tablespoons chili powder
- 4 pounds pork ribs

Instructions:

1. First of all, please make sure you have all the ingredients available. Preheat the oven to about 240 to 250°F.
2. Now mix together sea salt, paprika, black pepper, onion powder, chili powder, garlic

powder, cumin and cayenne pepper.

3. Now please rub the ribs with the spice mixture on both the sides.

4. This step is important. Place on a baking sheet, rib side down, & put into the oven.

5. Then cook properly for about 2 hours and 45 to 50 minutes, turning about every 15 to 20 minutes.

6. Broil the ribs for about 5 to 10 minutes to brown the meat side.

7. One thing remains to be done now. Take the ribs from the oven & let cool for about 5 to 10 minutes, then slice them.

8. Finally serve.

There it is.

Mighty Hearty Salmon Breakfast

Tasty dish just one step away!!

Ingredients:

- 2 eggs
- Salt and pepper to taste
- 2 cups of your choice of green leafy vegetable (spinach and green lettuce work well)
- Precooked and thinly sliced salmon (make sure to be aware of the sodium content)
- About 2.5 tablespoons butter
- 4 cherry tomatoes

Instructions:

1. First of all, please make sure you have all the ingredients available.

Now please place the butter in a saucepan & then turn the heat on.

2. Now while the butter is melting, place a pot full of water onto the stove & bring to a boil.
3. Once butter is melted, place the leafy green in the melted butter & toss until slightly limp.
4. This step is important. Then, set off to the side.
5. Then as water is coming to a boil, slice cherry tomatoes in half & follow the directions on the back of the salmon in order to prepare properly (some require heating & some can be eaten out of the package).
6. Now once the water is boiling, please crack the eggs into a ladle & then place the ladle slowly into the water for about 2 minutes.
7. Now quickly assemble. Place the leafy greens on a plate, then layer the salmon & tomatoes on top.

8. One thing remains to be done now. Place the poached eggs on top of everything, then sprinkle with salt & pepper to taste.
9. Finally enjoy!

I was waiting for this one.

Thanks for reading my book.